CANCER

DIET

COOKBOOK

2023 Latest Complete Cancer Diet Guide
Treatment And Anticancer Recipes,
Essential Nourishing Whole Food
1-20 Days Meal plan

Dr Buford L Brown

Table of contents

Introduction

In a world where the prevalence of cancer continues to rise, the quest for effective means of prevention and support has never been more urgent. The power of food as medicine has long been acknowledged, and in the realm of cancer care, it plays a pivotal role in promoting health, resilience, and overall well-being. "The Comprehensive Cancer Diet Cookbook" is a triumph in the pursuit of a holistic and integrative approach to cancer care, designed to be a guiding light for those on the challenging journey to recovery, healing, and prevention.

Within the pages of this extraordinary compendium, you will discover an extensive collection of recipes that seamlessly blend scientific insight with culinary creativity. From nutrient-packed smoothies to tantalising entrees and delectable desserts, this cookbook offers a treasure trove of delectable dishes carefully curated to nourish the body, mind, and soul. It is a testament to the adage that food is indeed thy medicine, offering not just sustenance, but a powerful ally in the battle against cancer.

What sets "The Comprehensive Cancer Diet Cookbook" apart is its commitment to evidence-based nutrition, drawing on the latest research and expert insights in the field. Each recipe is thoughtfully crafted to provide vital nutrients, antioxidants, and anti-inflammatory properties, aimed at fortifying the immune system, reducing inflammation, and encouraging the body's innate capacity to heal. Beyond the recipes, this book offers a comprehensive understanding of how dietary choices can impact cancer risk, treatment outcomes, and survivorship, with accessible explanations and expert guidance at every turn.

The authors, themselves seasoned experts in the realms of nutrition, oncology, and culinary arts, have joined forces to create a groundbreaking work that encompasses not just delicious and healthful recipes but a veritable roadmap for anyone touched by cancer. Their compassionate approach ensures that this cookbook is not just a culinary compendium but a beacon of hope and a source of empowerment for those seeking to regain control over their health.

"The Comprehensive Cancer Diet Cookbook" transcends the boundaries of a mere cookbook; it is an invitation to embark on a transformative culinary journey. Whether you are a cancer survivor, a dedicated caregiver, or someone looking to fortify their defences against this insidious disease, this book is an indispensable companion on the path to wellness. Prepare to be captivated by a world of flavours, rejuvenated by the nourishing power of food, and empowered to embrace a lifestyle that may not only enhance your resilience but also serve as a powerful force in your fight against cancer.

With its fusion of science, artistry, and unwavering dedication to promoting health and healing, this cookbook is poised to become an enduring masterpiece, a vital resource for those who seek not just to survive but to thrive in the face of cancer. Welcome to the world of "The Comprehensive Cancer Diet Cookbook," where every recipe is a celebration of life, a step towards recovery, and a testament to the remarkable potential of food as a healer.

Book Description

Are you or a loved one facing the battle against cancer and looking for ways to enhance your journey towards recovery?

Seeking the latest scientific insights on nutrition and its impact on cancer treatment in 2023?

Want to learn how the right diet can not only support but empower your body to fight this formidable foe?

Your answers lie within the pages of this transformative cookbook!

In this groundbreaking book, we draw on the most recent medical research of 2023 to provide you with a comprehensive guide on harnessing the power of nutrition to aid your fight against cancer. But this isn't just another cookbook - it's a beacon of hope for those navigating their way through this challenging path.

Discover a myriad of delectable, nutritious recipes tailored to nourish your body during your battle against cancer.

Learn how specific foods can help mitigate side effects of treatments and boost your immune system.

Understand the science behind each recipe, and how it can contribute to your overall well-being.

This book is your ultimate companion, answering crucial questions and providing much-needed guidance How can food play a pivotal role in your cancer journey?

☐ What cutting-edge 2023 medical insights are integrated into these recipes?

☐Why is proper nutrition essential during cancer treatment?

☐What recipes can alleviate symptoms and enhance your quality of life?

By the time you've explored these pages, you'll be equipped with the knowledge and culinary skills to help you, or your loved one, face cancer with resilience and optimism. Our mission is to empower you to take control of your health and well-being during these trying times.

No matter where you are in the cancer treatment process, choosing healthful foods is more important than ever. This Cancer Diet Cookbook is a useful resource for anyone undergoing cancer treatment and rehabilitation since it contains numerous recipes for quick and easy meals that are both nutritious and delicious.

This Cookbook features:

- Dozens of tasty, nutritious dishes----- Help control symptoms and enhance immunity both before and after treatment.

- Basics of cancer diet---Learn how cancer affects the body, how "cancer-fighting foods" can assist, and which foods to avoid.

- 28-Day Meal Plan---Accept a new, healthier eating style that is ideal for patients.

- Premium Full Color Pictures--- So that you won't feel bored while cooking, but will have your appetite whetted by the pictures.l

With each page you turn, you'll find renewed hope, practical advice, and a wealth of delicious recipes that make the cancer journey more manageable and even enjoyable. This cookbook is not just about fighting cancer; it's about thriving through nourishment, knowledge, and unwavering support.

Take the first step towards a healthier, brighter future. Order your copy of the "Cancer Diet Cookbook" today and let the healing power of food guide your path to recovery. Your journey starts here!

Chapter One

What is Cancer

Cancer, often referred to as the "Emperor of All Maladies," is a formidable adversary that has plagued humanity for centuries. It is a multifaceted and relentless disease that manifests when the intricate machinery of the human body goes awry. To comprehend the profound impact of cancer on our lives and the astounding strides made in understanding, treating, and supporting those affected, we must delve into its basis, explore the diverse treatment modalities, consider the role of clinical trials, and highlight the essential support systems in place.

The Basis of Cancer: A Cellular Rebellion

At its core, cancer is a disease of uncontrolled cell growth. Normal, healthy cells within the human body follow a well-orchestrated pattern of growth, division, and death. However, when certain genetic mutations or external factors disrupt this balance, a single cell may transform into a malignant entity, capable of evading the body's regulatory mechanisms. This cellular rebellion is the fundamental basis of cancer.

Cancer is not a single disease but rather a group of diseases. It can originate in any tissue or organ, and the type of cancer is typically named after the tissue where it begins. Common forms include breast cancer, lung cancer, and colon cancer, each with distinct characteristics and behaviours.

Proper Treatments: A Multifaceted Approach

The fight against cancer involves an arsenal of treatments, tailored to the specific type and stage of the disease. The primary modalities include surgery, chemotherapy, radiation therapy, immunotherapy, targeted therapy, and hormone therapy. These treatments aim to eradicate or control the cancerous cells while minimising damage to healthy tissues.

Surgery, often the first line of defence, involves the removal of cancerous growths. Chemotherapy and radiation therapy employ the use of chemicals and high-energy radiation to destroy cancer cells. Immunotherapy enhances the body's immune system to recognize and attack cancer cells. Targeted therapy focuses on specific molecular abnormalities within cancer cells, while hormone therapy is effective against hormone-related cancers, such as breast and prostate cancer.

Clinical Trials: Pioneering the Future of Cancer Care

Clinical trials are the lifeblood of cancer research and treatment. They are a critical bridge between laboratory discoveries and real-world applications. These trials are designed to evaluate the safety and effectiveness of new treatments, as well as to identify better ways to diagnose, prevent, and manage cancer. Engaging in a clinical trial can be a courageous step for both patients and researchers, as it represents a quest for innovation and progress in the realm of cancer care.

Support Groups: The Power of Community

Coping with cancer can be emotionally, mentally, and physically challenging. To address these challenges, support groups have emerged as invaluable resources. These groups offer a sense of community, understanding, and shared experiences that can be profoundly comforting for cancer patients and their loved ones. Support groups provide an environment where individuals can discuss their fears, uncertainties, and triumphs, while also receiving practical advice and emotional encouragement.

In addition to peer-led support groups, professional counseling and therapy services are also available, offering specialised guidance in managing the psychological and emotional toll that cancer can bring.

Note, cancer is a complex and pervasive disease that strikes at the very essence of our being. Its basis in cellular rebellion has driven relentless research efforts to develop a range of treatments, including surgery, chemotherapy, radiation therapy, immunotherapy, targeted therapy, and hormone therapy. Clinical trials stand as beacons of hope, leading us toward the future of cancer care. Meanwhile, support groups and professional services provide the vital emotional and psychological sustenance needed by patients and their families. As science and medicine continue to advance, the understanding, treatment, and support for those affected by cancer will undoubtedly become even more impressive and effective, ultimately bringing us closer to conquering the Emperor of All Maladies.

Chapter Two

Cancer Diet

A cancer diagnosis can be a life-altering moment, and it often prompts individuals to reevaluate many aspects of their lives, including their diet. The relationship between cancer and diet is a complex one, and while a specific diet may not be a cure, it can play a significant role in supporting overall health and well-being during cancer treatment and recovery. In this comprehensive exploration of the cancer diet, we will delve into some of the dietary principles and recipes that have shown promise in helping individuals on their journey to better health.

1.Anti-Inflammatory Foods:

Inflammation is closely linked to cancer development and progression. A diet rich in anti-inflammatory foods can help combat this process. Incorporating ingredients such as turmeric, ginger, and green tea can reduce inflammation. A classic recipe to consider is a turmeric-infused lentil soup, which offers both comfort and healing benefits.

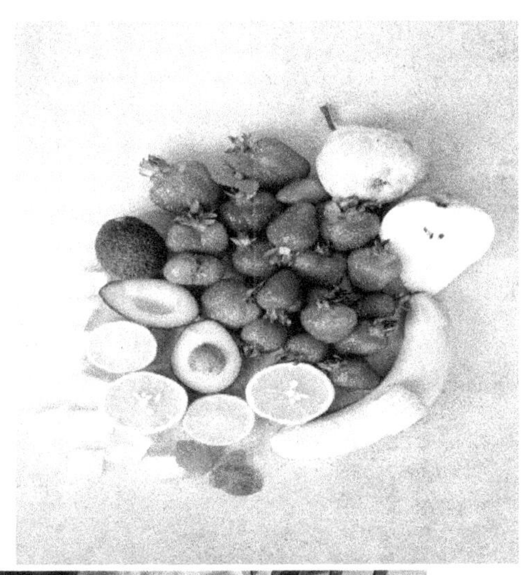

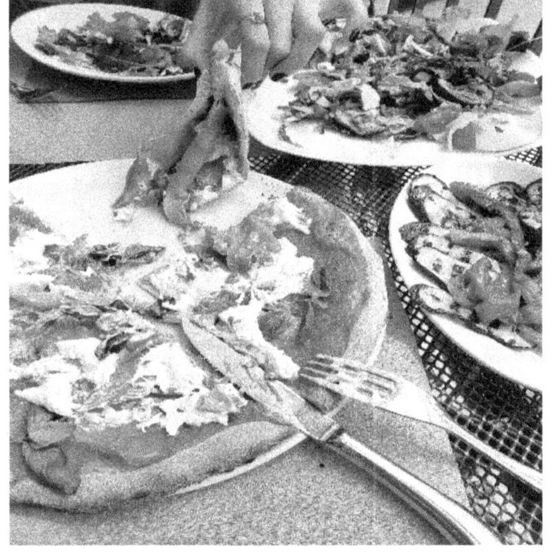

2.Cruciferous Vegetables:

Cruciferous vegetables like broccoli, cauliflower, kale, and Brussels sprouts are packed with cancer-fighting compounds. These veggies contain sulforaphane, a natural plant compound that has been found to have potential anti-cancer properties. A delightful recipe featuring these vegetables is a roasted broccoli and cauliflower salad, paired with a lemon-tahini dressing.

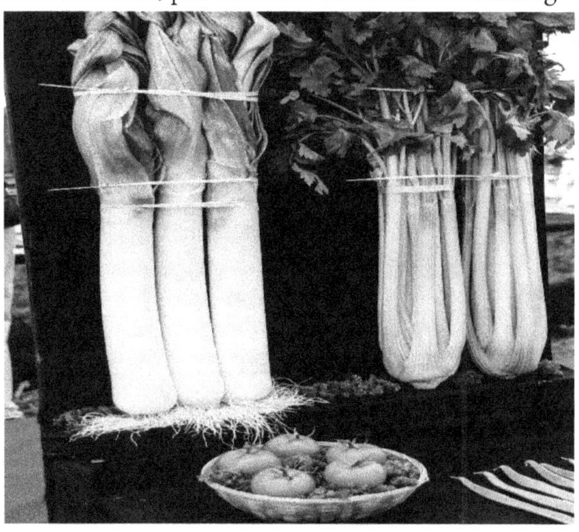

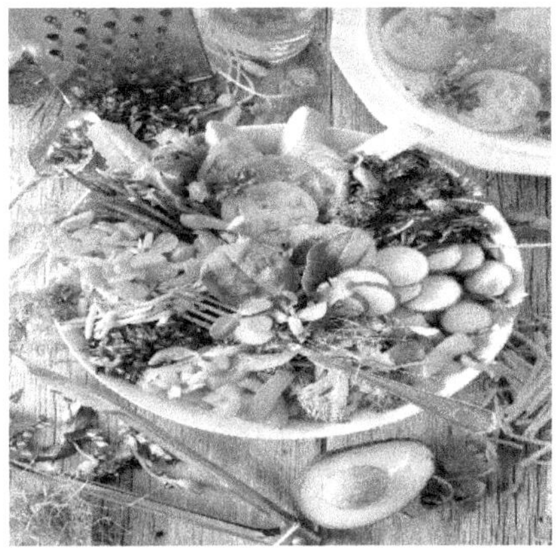

3.Fibre-Rich Foods:

Fibre is essential for digestive health and can help reduce the risk of certain cancers. Whole grains, legumes, and fruits are excellent sources of dietary fibre. A hearty and satisfying recipe could be a quinoa and black bean bowl topped with a colourful array of fruits and vegetables.

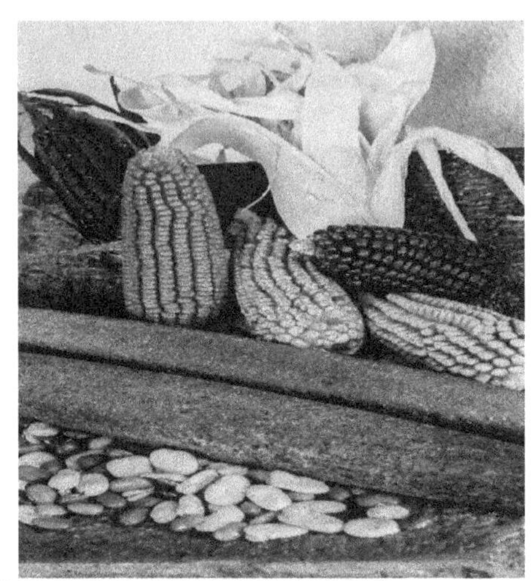

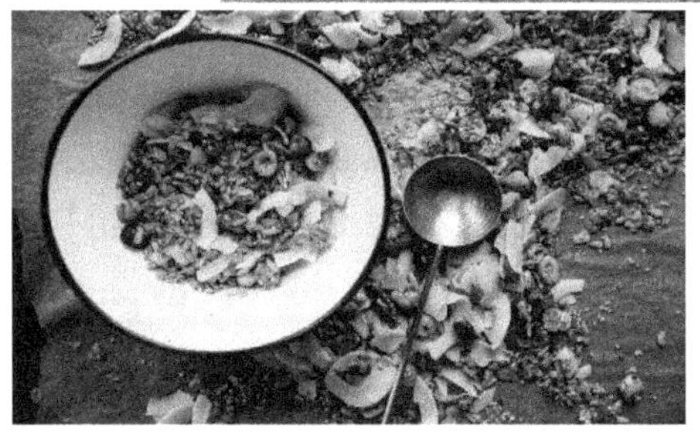

4. Omega-3 Fatty Acids:

Omega-3 fatty acids, found in fatty fish like salmon, flaxseeds, and walnuts, have demonstrated potential in reducing inflammation and protecting against cancer. A mouthwatering recipe could be a grilled salmon fillet served with a side of quinoa and roasted asparagus.

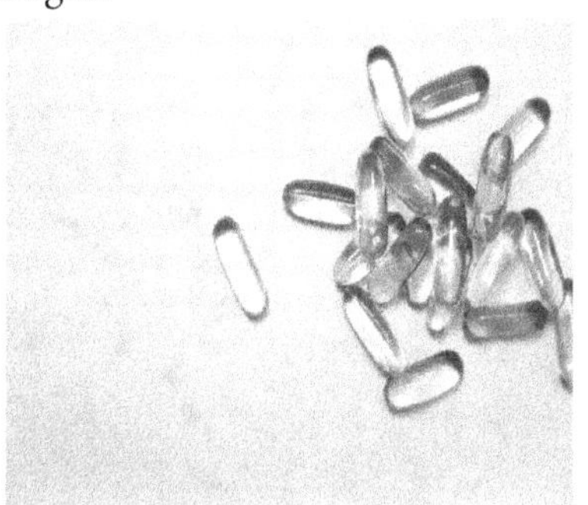

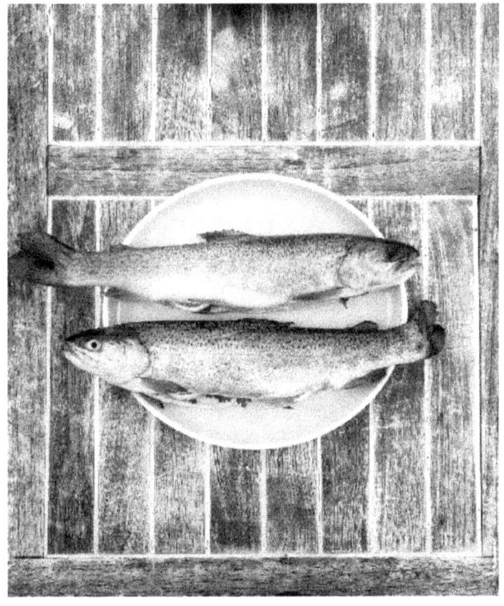

5. Plant-Based Diet:

A plant-based diet, characterised by an abundance of fruits, vegetables, nuts, and seeds, can be highly beneficial for cancer patients. A simple yet delectable recipe is a Mediterranean-style salad with mixed greens, olives, and a zesty hummus dressing.

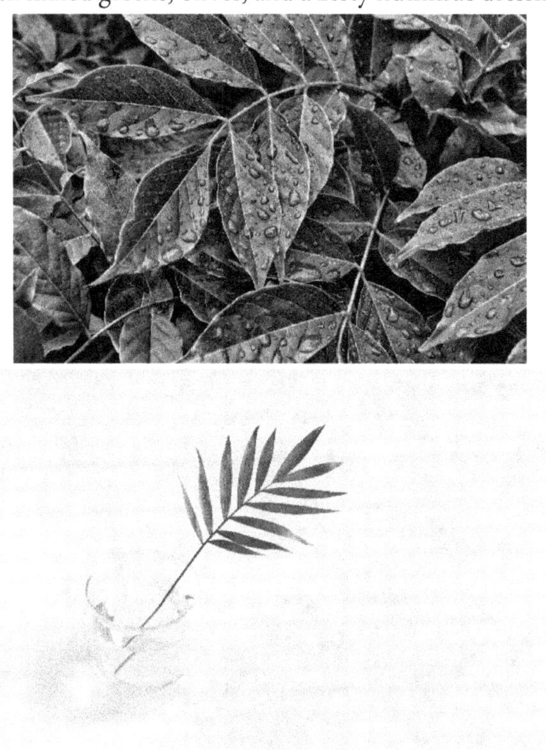

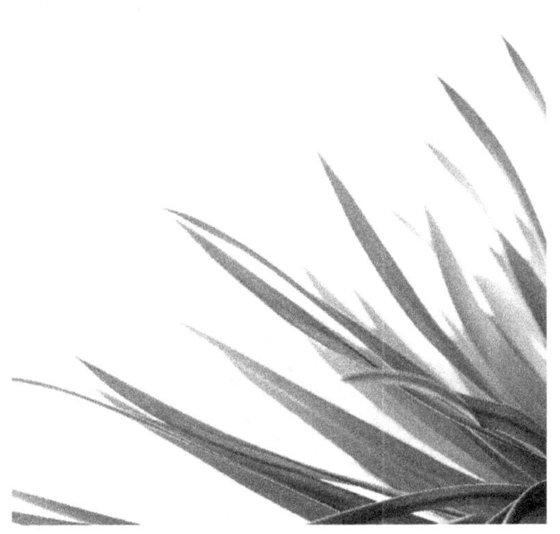

6. Herbal Teas:

Certain herbal teas, such as green tea and chamomile, have antioxidant properties that may help protect cells from damage. Sipping on a warm cup of green tea or enjoying a calming chamomile infusion can be a soothing addition to the daily routine.

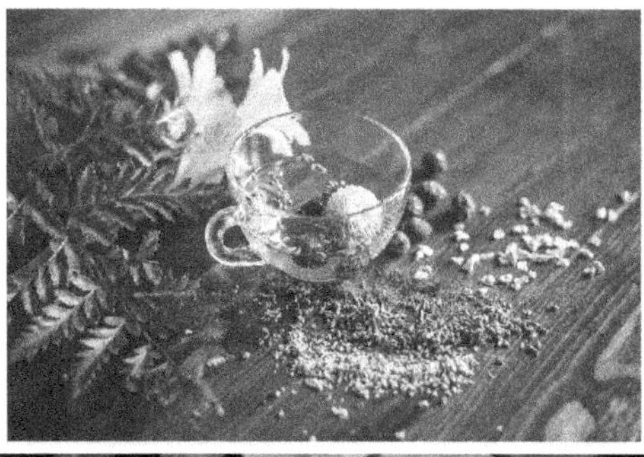

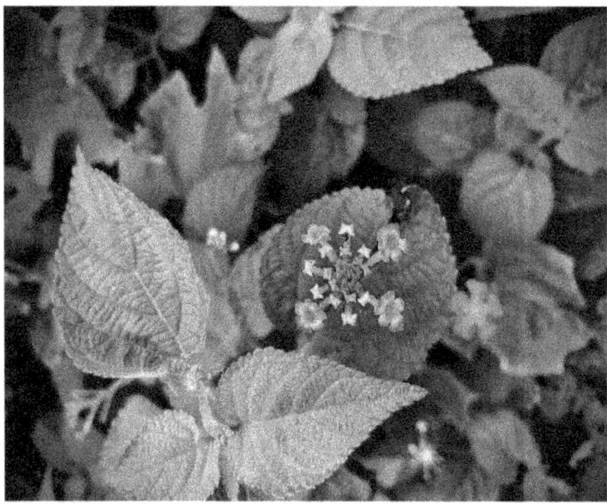

7. Hydration:

Staying well-hydrated is crucial during cancer treatment. Adequate water intake supports the body's functions and helps manage side effects like fatigue and nausea. A pitcher of infused water with slices of cucumber, lemon, and mint can make hydration more appealing.

While these dietary principles and recipes can contribute to a healthier lifestyle during cancer treatment, it's essential to remember that they are not a substitute for medical advice or treatment. Always consult with a healthcare professional or a registered dietitian when making significant dietary changes, especially when managing a cancer diagnosis.

8.Exercise

Exercise is not only a cornerstone of physical fitness but also an invaluable ally in the battle against cancer. The idea that a physically active lifestyle can help reduce the risk of cancer and aid in cancer management has gained significant traction in recent years. In this extensive exploration, we will delve into the impressive ways in which exercise contributes to the prevention and management of various types of cancer.

1.Aerobic Exercises: The benefits of aerobic exercises such as running, swimming, and cycling are multifaceted. These exercises stimulate the cardiovascular system, increase oxygen supply, and improve overall circulation. They also promote the body's natural detoxification process, which can help reduce the risk of certain types of cancer, such as lung, colon, and breast cancer

2.Strength Training: Building lean muscle mass through strength training exercises like weightlifting can be a powerful ally in the fight against cancer. Muscle tissues can aid in metabolising and using insulin more effectively, reducing the risk of cancers like pancreatic cancer. Moreover, muscle strength can improve balance and mobility, reducing the risk of falls in older individuals.

Yoga: The practice of yoga not only enhances flexibility and mental well-being but can also contribute to cancer prevention. The stress-reducing and relaxation benefits of yoga may help to regulate the stress hormone cortisol, which, when chronically elevated, is associated with an increased risk of various cancers.

Pilates: Pilates exercises focus on core strength, posture, and flexibility. These exercises can aid in the management of cancer-related fatigue and discomfort. For cancer survivors, Pilates can be a valuable tool in restoring physical function and improving overall quality of life.

Tai Chi: Tai Chi is a low-impact, slow-motion exercise that combines gentle movements and deep breathing. Studies suggest that Tai Chi can be particularly beneficial for breast cancer survivors, helping with balance, coordination, and reducing the severity of lymphedema.

High-Intensity Interval Training (HIIT):

HIIT workouts involve short bursts of intense activity followed by brief rest periods. This type of exercise can be time-efficient and effective in reducing body fat, which, in turn, may lower the risk of obesity-related cancers like endometrial and colorectal cancer.

Mindful Walking: Even something as simple as regular, brisk walking can have a profound impact on cancer risk. Walking stimulates the lymphatic system, helping to remove waste and toxins from the body. Additionally, regular walking can promote healthy weight maintenance, which is a key factor in cancer prevention.

Swimming: Swimming is a full-body workout that is gentle on the joints. It can be especially beneficial for people undergoing cancer treatment, as it provides both cardiovascular and muscular benefits while reducing the impact on the body. Swimming can help manage side effects of cancer treatments like fatigue and muscle weakness.

Dance Therapy: Dancing isn't just a form of exercise; it's also a powerful emotional outlet. Dance therapy can help cancer patients and survivors cope with stress and anxiety. The expressive nature of dance can boost mental well-being and improve overall quality of life.

Meditation: While not a physical exercise in the traditional sense, meditation is a vital component of cancer care. Reducing stress through meditation can help the immune system function optimally, aiding in cancer prevention and recovery.

Exercise serves as a multifaceted weapon against cancer, with its ability to reduce cancer risk, improve treatment outcomes, and enhance the overall well-being of cancer survivors. It's crucial to note that the benefits of exercise may vary depending on the type of cancer, the stage of the disease, and individual health conditions. Therefore, consultation with a healthcare provider is advised to develop a tailored exercise plan that is safe and effective for each person's unique circumstances. By incorporating a variety of exercises into one's routine, individuals can harness the impressive benefits that physical activity offers in the fight against cancer.

The relationship between cancer and diet is a multifaceted one. A well-balanced and thoughtfully crafted diet can provide valuable support during cancer treatment and recovery. By incorporating anti-inflammatory foods, cruciferous vegetables, fibre-rich options, omega-3 fatty acids, and embracing a plant-based approach, individuals can empower themselves with a more holistic approach to healing and overall well-being. Remember, a healthy diet is just one piece of the puzzle, and it should be part of a broader strategy that includes medical treatment, emotional support, and a positive mindset.

Chapter Three

Special Meals

In the intricate tapestry of cancer care, the role of nutrition emerges as a powerful ally in fostering strength and resilience. Tailoring a diet to meet the unique needs of cancer patients involves a thoughtful selection of foods renowned for their healing properties.

Turmeric:Harnessing the anti-inflammatory prowess of curcumin, turmeric stands as a culinary titan. Its potential to alleviate inflammation may aid in mitigating the side effects of cancer treatments, offering a flavorful addition to dishes.

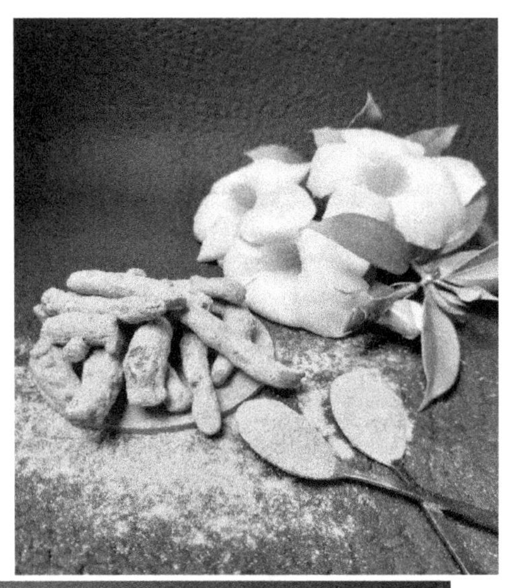

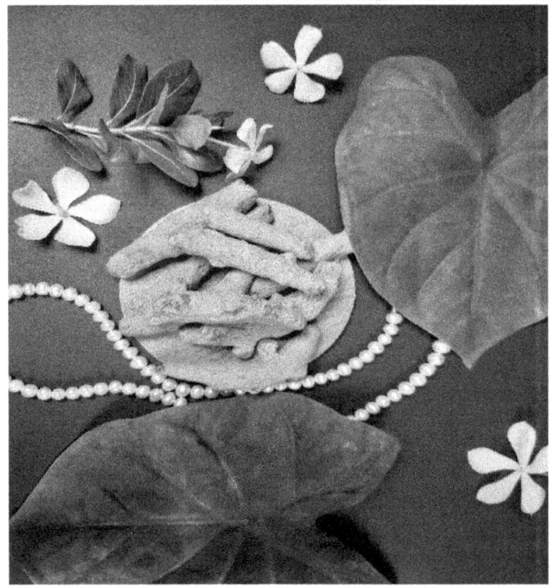

Cruciferous Vegetables:

Broccoli, kale, and cauliflower, among others, contribute to the arsenal of cancer-fighting foods. Rich in antioxidants and phytochemicals, these cruciferous gems bolster the body's defence mechanisms.

Berries:

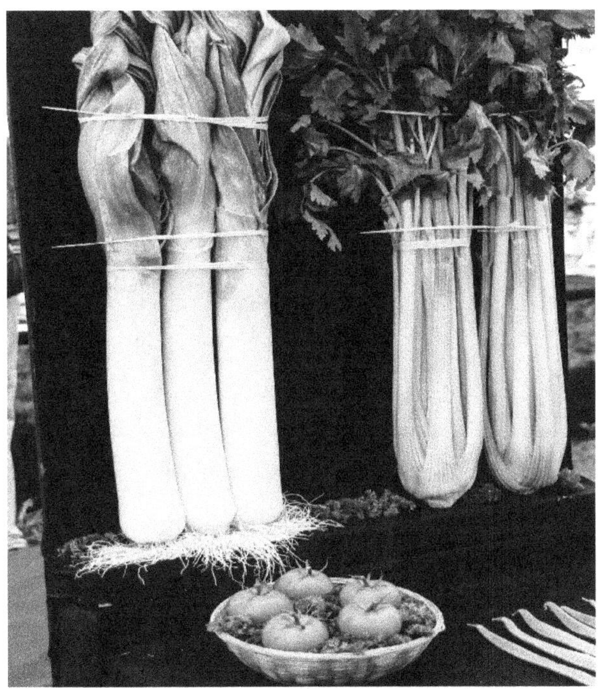

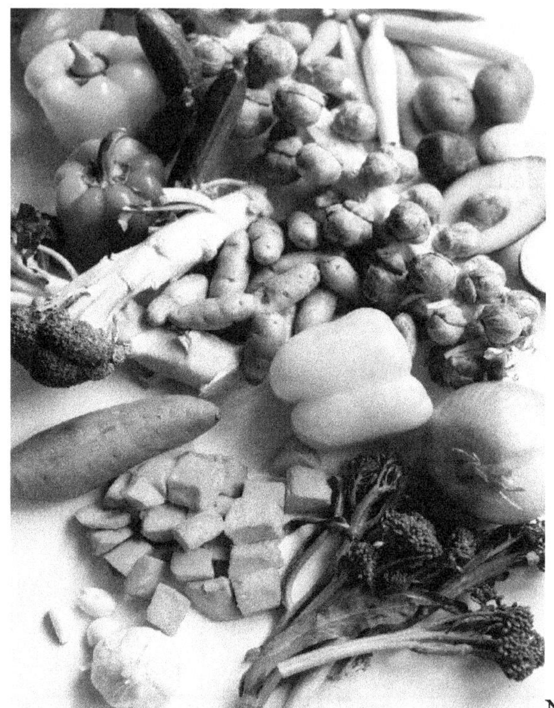

Nature's sweet antidote, berries boast a vibrant spectrum of antioxidants. Their role in reducing oxidative stress is pivotal, potentially enhancing the body's ability to combat the challenges posed by chance

Fatty Fish:

Laden with omega-3 fatty acids, fish like salmon and mackerel offer a dual benefit—supporting cardiovascular health and exhibiting potential anti-cancer properties.

Ginger:

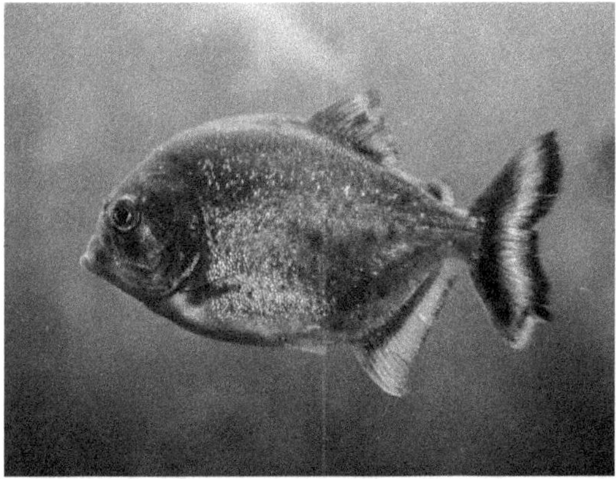

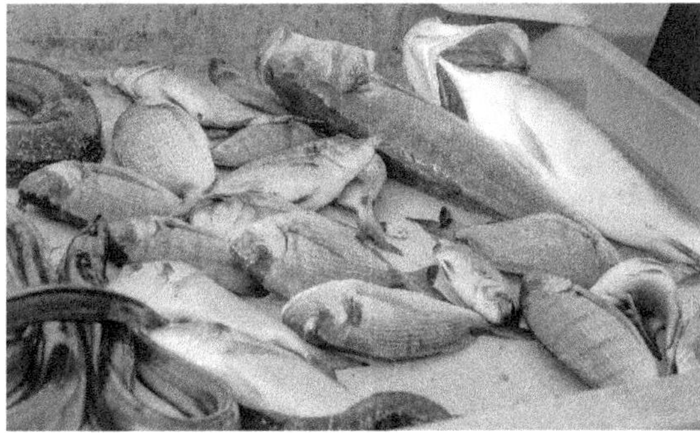

Celebrated for its anti-nausea properties, ginger becomes a soothing companion for cancer patients navigating the often turbulent seas of treatment. Its aromatic presence adds depth to both meals and relief.

Leafy Greens:

Spinach, kale, and Swiss chard form a verdant symphony of nutrients. Packed with vitamins, minerals, and fibre, they contribute to overall well-being and vitality during the recovery journey.

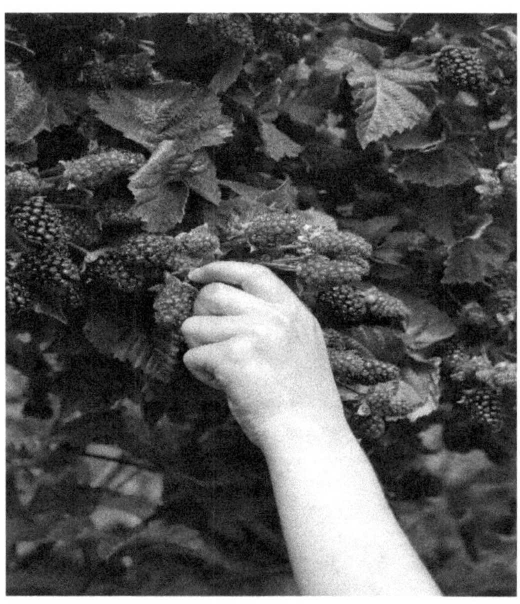

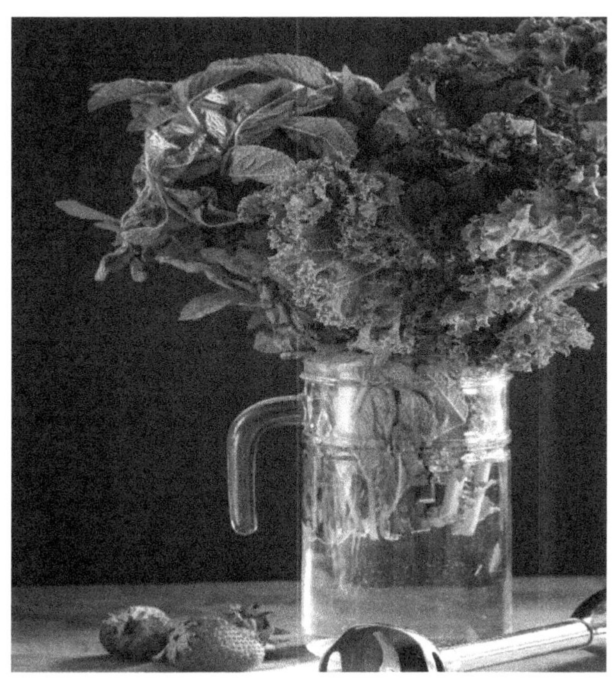

Green Tea:

Beyond a refreshing beverage, green tea holds catechins, compounds with potential cancer-fighting properties. Sipping on this elixir provides hydration intertwined with a dash of wellness

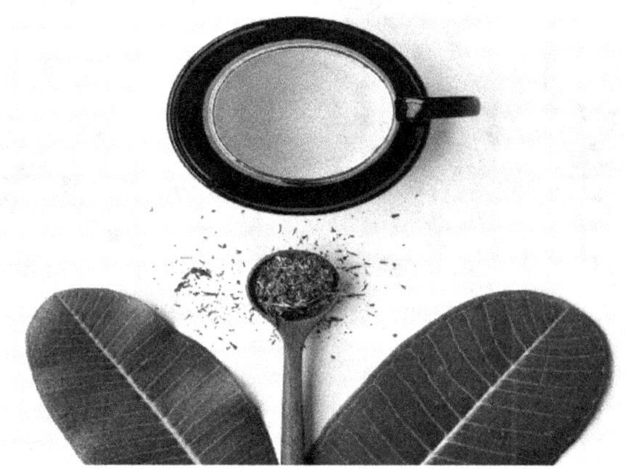

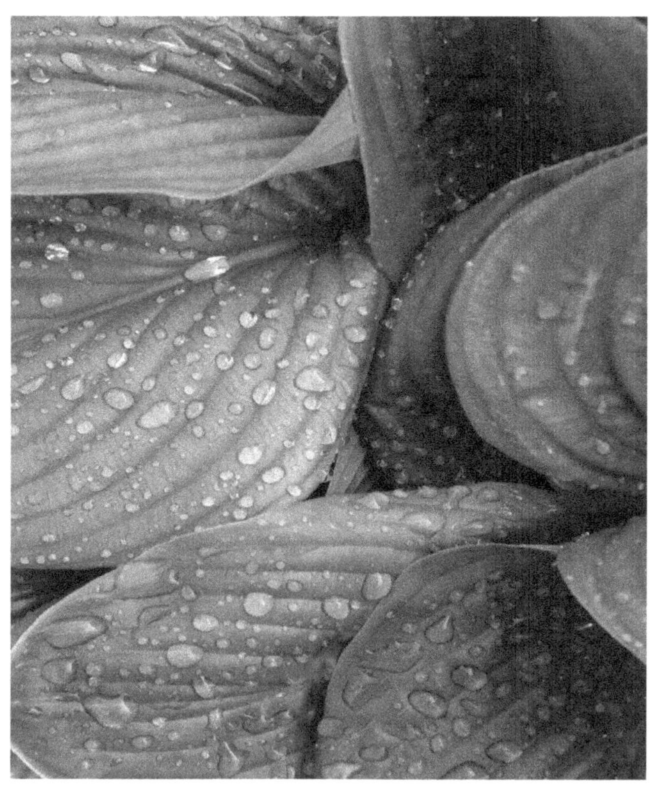

Quinoa:

As a complete protein source, quinoa offers a nutritional lifeline, supporting muscle maintenance and repair—an invaluable asset in the face of the physical demands associated with cancer treatments.

In navigating the labyrinth of dietary choices, the synergy of these foods forms a nourishing narrative. Crafting meals that blend flavour with therapeutic benefits becomes a culinary act of compassion, empowering cancer patients on their path to healing.

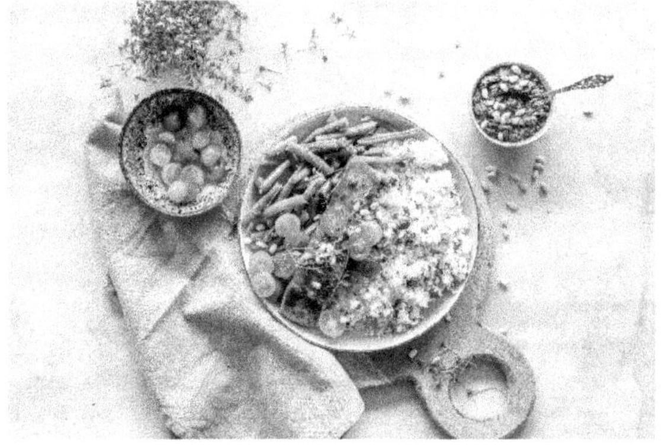

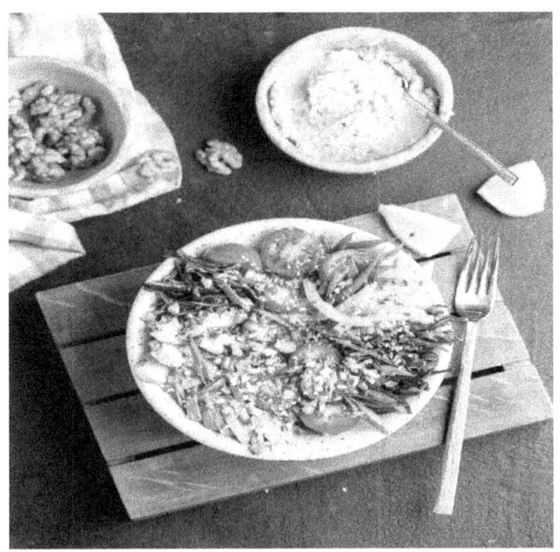

Chapter Four

Antioxidant Rich Recipes For Boosting Immunity

Boosting immunity through antioxidant-rich recipes is not only a delicious endeavour but also a proactive approach to overall well-being. These recipes are not just meals; they are a celebration of vibrant flavours and health benefits.

1. Berry Blast Smoothie:

Start your day with a burst of antioxidants by blending a mix of blueberries, strawberries, and raspberries. Add a dollop of Greek yoghourts for probiotics and a handful of spinach for an extra nutrient kick.

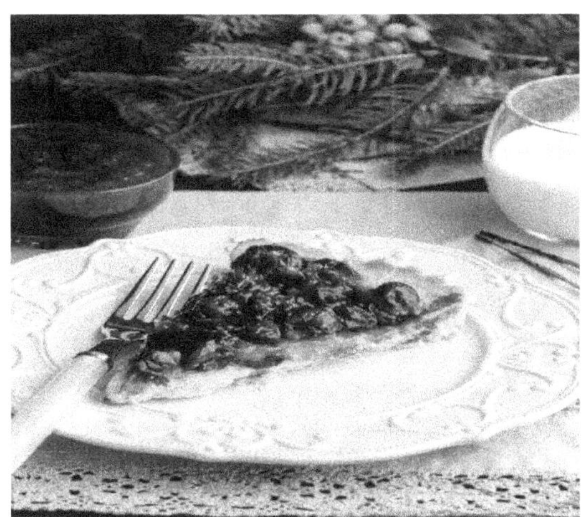

2. Quinoa Salad with Pomegranate:

Combine the protein-packed quinoa with the antioxidant power of pomegranate seeds. Toss in some chopped cucumber, mint, and feta cheese for a refreshing and immunity-boosting salad.

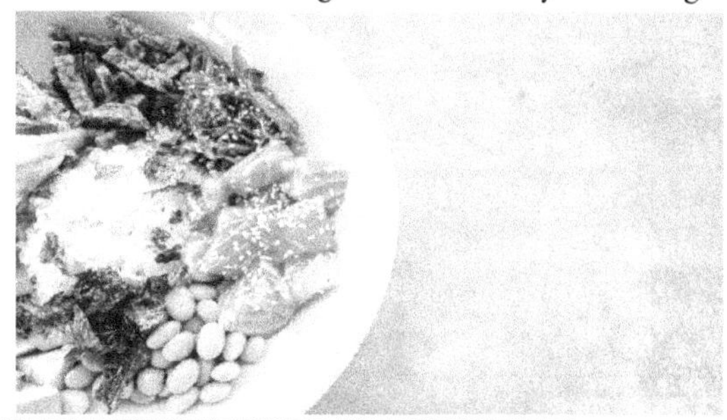

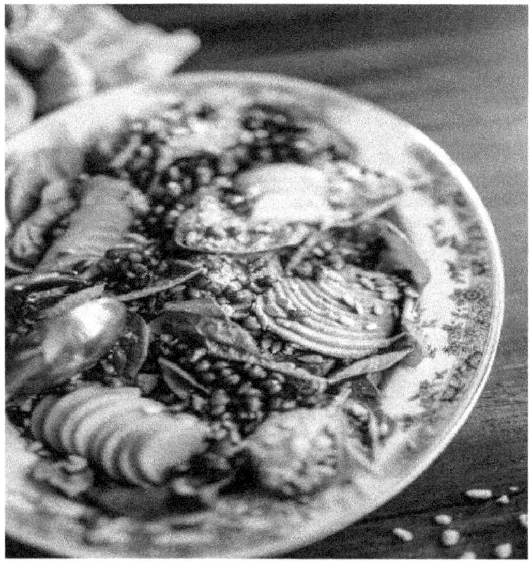

3. Turmeric-Ginger Infused Tea:

Harness the anti-inflammatory properties of turmeric and ginger by brewing a comforting tea. Add a dash of honey for sweetness and a squeeze of lemon for a vitamin C boost.

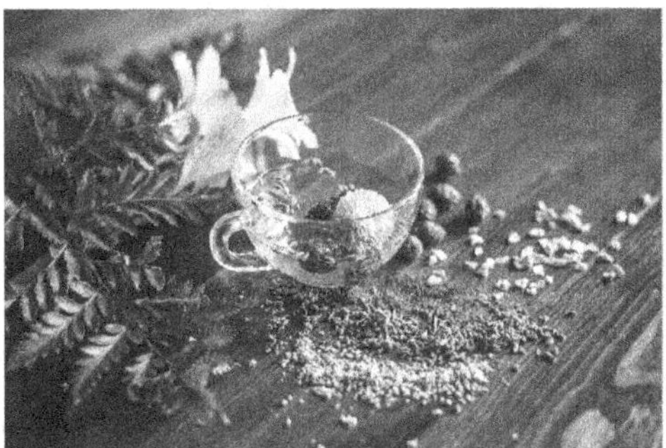

4. Roasted Vegetable Medley:

Create a colorful plate of antioxidants by roasting a variety of vegetables such as bell peppers, carrots, and broccoli. Drizzle with olive oil and sprinkle with herbs for a flavorful immune-boosting side dish.

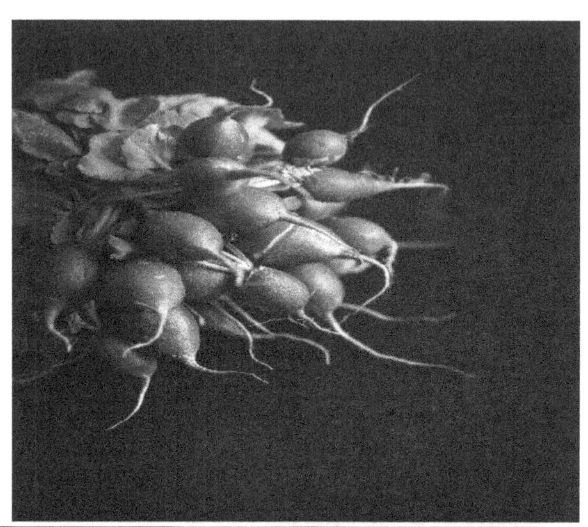

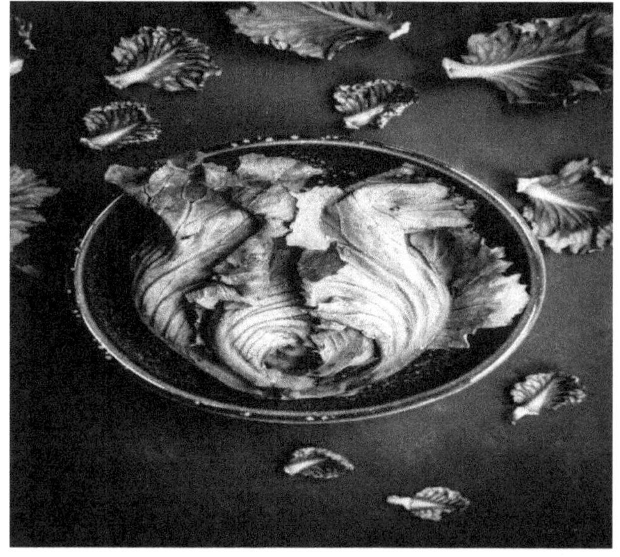

5. Garlic-Lemon Salmon:

Grill or bake salmon with a marinade of minced garlic, lemon juice, and herbs. The combination not only enhances the taste but also provides a dose of antioxidants and omega-3 fatty acids.

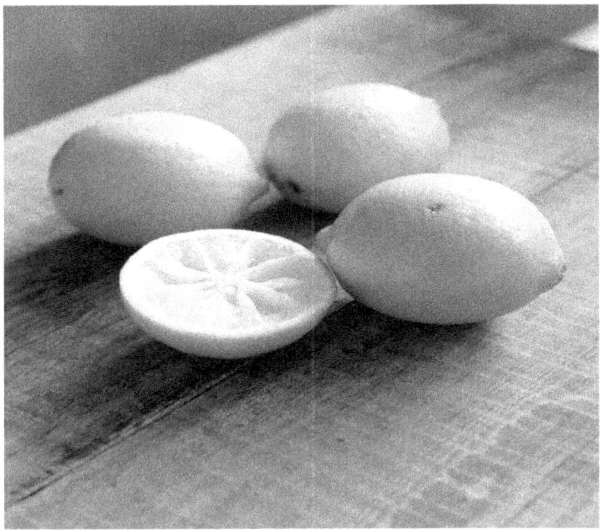

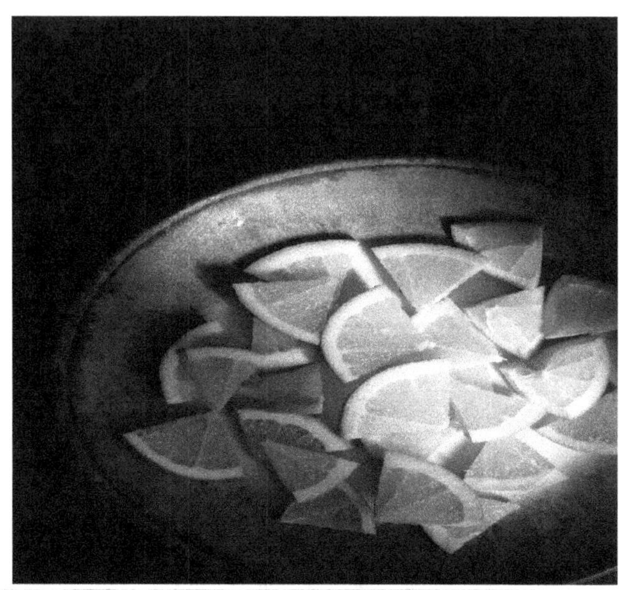

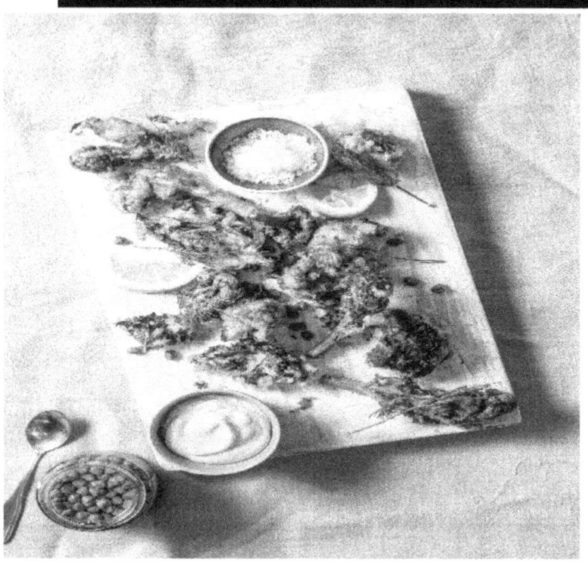

6. Spinach and Kale Stuffed Chicken Breast:

Prepare a nutrient-rich entrée by stuffing chicken breasts with a mixture of sautéed spinach, kale, and garlic. Bake until golden brown for a dish that's high in vitamins and minerals.

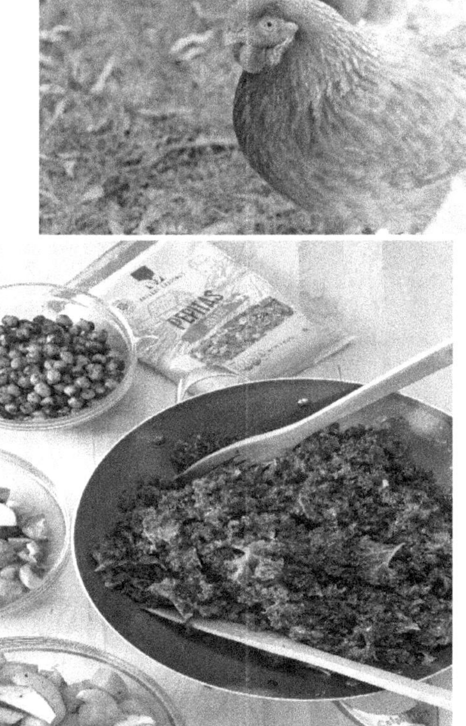

7. Dark Chocolate-Berry Parfait:

Indulge your sweet tooth with a guilt-free dessert. Layer dark chocolate shavings with a mix of antioxidant-rich berries and a dollop of Greek yogurt for a decadent yet healthy treat.

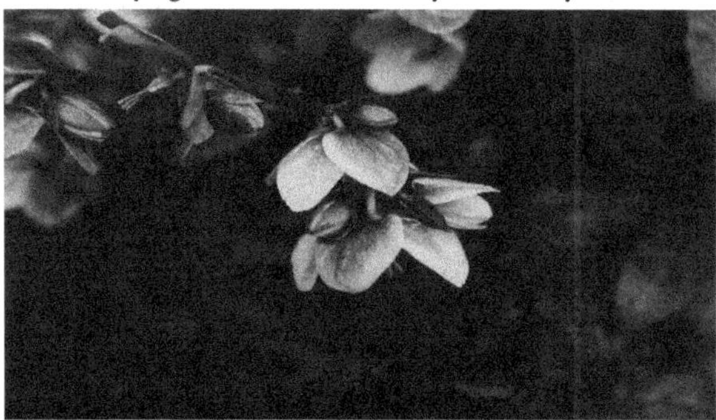

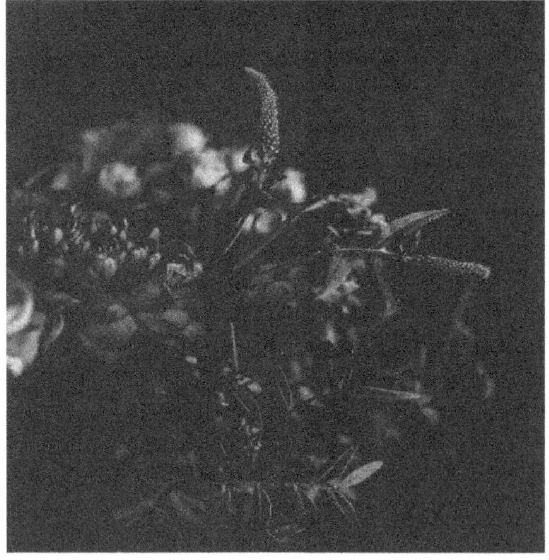

8. Green Tea Chia Pudding:

Combine the antioxidant properties of green tea with the nutritional goodness of chia seeds. Mix them with almond milk and let it set overnight for a delightful and immune-boosting breakfast.

9. Citrus-Marinated Chicken Skewers:

Marinate chicken chunks in a zesty mix of citrus juices, garlic, and herbs before grilling. The vitamin C from the citrus fruits adds a refreshing twist and supports your immune system.

10. Tomato Basil Quinoa Bowl:

Create a simple yet flavorful bowl by combining cooked quinoa with fresh tomatoes, basil, and a drizzle of balsamic glaze. This recipe is not only rich in antioxidants but also a delightful symphony of tastes.

Incorporating these antioxidant-rich recipes into your diet not only elevates your culinary experience but also contributes to a robust immune system. Embrace the vibrant colors and diverse flavors, and let your journey to better health be a delicious one.

Chapter Five

Incorporating more vegetables into your diet

The Power of a Plant-Forward Plate

In the realm of cancer-fighting nutrition, vegetables emerge as the unsung heroes, wielding an arsenal of vitamins, minerals, antioxidants, and phytochemicals. Our journey begins by unraveling the science behind these potent plant-based warriors, revealing how they collaborate to fortify your body's defenses against the formidable adversary that is cancer.

A Palette of Phytonutrients

Dive deep into the vibrant spectrum of phytonutrients found in vegetables, each contributing its unique hue and health benefits. From the lycopene-rich reds to the cruciferous greens, we explore the kaleidoscope of colors that not only adds visual appeal to your plate but also serves as a potent shield against oxidative stress and inflammation.

Crafting Culinary Masterpieces

Embark on a culinary adventure as we transform vegetables into delectable masterpieces that delight the senses. From roasted root vegetables drizzled with savory herb-infused oils to vibrant salads bursting with a symphony of textures, these recipes are meticulously crafted to elevate the dining experience while championing the cause of well-being.

The Dance of Flavors and Textures

Discover the art of balancing flavors and textures as we explore the versatility of vegetables. From the subtle crunch of julienned carrots to the creamy richness of roasted sweet potatoes, learn how to orchestrate a culinary dance that not only satisfies your palate but also nurtures your body at its core.

A Garden of Healing Herbs and Spices

Delve into the world of healing herbs and spices that complement the vegetable-rich foundation of your cancer-fighting diet. Uncover the medicinal properties of turmeric, the aromatic embrace of basil, and the soothing notes of mint as we infuse your culinary creations with a therapeutic touch.

Chapter Six

Protein packed meals for strength and recovery

In the realm of fitness and well-being, the significance of protein-packed meals for strength and recovery stands as an undeniable cornerstone. A carefully crafted diet enriched with high-protein sources not only fuels the body's muscular development but also plays a pivotal role in post-exertion recuperation. However, in the pursuit of this nutritional nirvana, individuals often encounter a myriad of challenges.

One of the foremost predicaments faced by fitness enthusiasts is the bewildering array of protein options available. From plant-based alternatives like tofu and quinoa to animal-derived powerhouses like chicken and salmon, navigating this labyrinthine selection can be overwhelming. The task is further complicated by dietary restrictions and preferences, as some may opt for vegetarian or vegan paths while others embrace carnivorous inclinations.

Yet, beyond the tantalizing array of choices, the issue of adequate protein intake often becomes a stumbling block. Many individuals, whether due to time constraints or misinformation, fall prey to insufficient protein consumption, hindering their progress in the gym and impeding the body's ability to recover effectively. The consequences of such negligence extend beyond the realms of muscle development, impacting overall performance and leaving individuals susceptible to prolonged fatigue and increased susceptibility to injuries.

In the landscape of protein-packed meals, the timing of consumption emerges as a critical factor. The elusive golden window post-workout demands attention, with experts emphasizing the importance of replenishing protein stores promptly to maximize the benefits of exercise. Failing to capitalize on this temporal window can result in diminished gains, sluggish recovery, and the frustrating sense of plateau that many fitness enthusiasts dread.

However, the challenges don't end there. Despite the growing awareness of the significance of protein in strength and recovery, misconceptions linger. The misguided fear of protein-induced kidney damage and the misconception that protein supplements are reserved solely for bodybuilders are but a few myths that permeate the fitness landscape, potentially deterring individuals from optimizing their nutrition for peak performance.

Amidst these challenges, a silver lining exists – a myriad of delectable and protein-rich culinary creations that not only satisfy the taste buds but also cater to the body's nutritional needs. From hearty lentil stews and tempeh stir-fries to succulent grilled chicken and salmon filets, the options are as diverse as they are nutritious. The fusion of flavors and textures in these protein-packed masterpieces transforms the seemingly mundane act of eating into a symphony of nourishment and satisfaction.

The journey towards harnessing the power of protein for strength and recovery is not without its trials and tribulations. The path is laden with the complexities of choice, the specter of inadequate intake, and the nuances of timing. Yet, it is within this labyrinth of challenges that the key to unlocking one's true physical potential resides. With knowledge as a guide and a palate tuned to the symphony of protein-rich delights, individuals can navigate these challenges, sculpting not just their bodies but a lifestyle that harmonizes with the pursuit of strength, vitality, and enduring wellness.

Chapter Seven

Healthy fats and Omega 3s :

Embracing a culinary paradigm that champions sources of healthy fats, such as avocados, nuts, and olive oil, introduces a palatable symphony of taste and nourishment. These nutrient-dense options harbor monounsaturated and polyunsaturated fats, which have been associated with lower inflammation levels – a key consideration in the context of cancer, where chronic inflammation can contribute to disease progression.

Enter Omega-3 fatty acids, the unsung heroes of the culinary landscape. Abundantly found in fatty fish like salmon, mackerel, and sardines, as well as in flaxseeds and walnuts, Omega-3s are renowned for their anti-inflammatory properties. Their inclusion in a cancer-focused diet not only imparts a delectable zest but also fosters an environment less conducive to the development and proliferation of cancer cells.

Moreover, the synergistic interplay between these healthy fats and Omega-3s extends beyond taste and inflammation control. These nutritional powerhouses have been linked to cellular health, immune system modulation, and even potential benefits in cancer treatment support. By incorporating a diverse array of ingredients rich in these vital nutrients, the Cancer Diet Cookbook emerges not merely as a collection of recipes but as a culinary compendium that actively engages with the intricacies of health and wellbeing.

In summary, the judicious integration of healthy fats and Omega-3s in the Cancer Diet Cookbook serves as a testament to the transformative potential of nutrition. Through this gastronomic exploration, readers embark on a journey where each dish becomes a nourishing agent, contributing not only to the pleasure of the palate but also to the broader canvas of a health-conscious lifestyle.

Chapter Eight

Training your diet to specific cancer types

In the realm of health and nutrition, a groundbreaking frontier is emerging—one that delves into the intricate relationship between diet and specific cancer types. As we navigate the labyrinth of medical science, the concept of training our diets to address distinct cancers is gaining momentum, offering a beacon of hope in the fight against this formidable adversary.

Breast Cancer and the Power of Phytoestrogens:

For those grappling with the specter of breast cancer, a diet rich in phytoestrogens takes center stage. Embracing the goodness of foods like flaxseeds, soy, and lentils can provide a potent arsenal. These compounds, found in plant-based sources, mimic the action of estrogen in the body, potentially reducing the risk and progression of breast cancer.

Colorectal Cancer and the Fiber Connection:

The battle against colorectal cancer often calls for a strategic alliance with fiber-rich foods. Whole grains, fruits, and vegetables become the heroes of this dietary saga, wielding their power to promote digestive health and thwart the onset of colorectal malignancies. Fiber acts as a guardian, aiding in the removal of potentially harmful substances from the body.

Prostate Cancer and the Lycopene Shield:

In the realm of prostate health, lycopene emerges as a formidable ally. This antioxidant, prevalent in tomatoes, watermelon, and guavas, has been linked to a potential reduction in prostate cancer risk. Including these vibrant, lycopene-rich foods in one's diet serves as a shield, fortifying the body against the challenges posed by prostate malignancies.

Lung Cancer and the Cruciferous Crusade:

As we confront the complexities of lung cancer, the cruciferous vegetables step into the limelight. Broccoli, kale, and Brussels sprouts, armed with their arsenal of anti-cancer compounds, embark on a crusade against lung carcinogens. Sulforaphane, a key player in this green battalion, demonstrates promising anti-cancer properties, offering a glimmer of hope in the battle against lung cancer.

Pancreatic Cancer and the Turmeric Touch:

The enigmatic and often elusive pancreatic cancer invites a culinary companion: turmeric. Curcumin, the active ingredient in turmeric, exhibits anti-inflammatory and anti-cancer properties. This golden spice, woven into the fabric of cuisines for centuries, takes on a new role as a potential protector against pancreatic malignancies, urging us to embrace its vibrant hue for the sake of our health.

As we tailor our diets to specific cancer types, a symphony of flavors and nutrients becomes our armor against an insidious foe. This personalized approach not only signifies a revolution in cancer prevention but also celebrates the resilience of the human spirit, finding strength and healing in the very sustenance that fuels our existence. In the realm of nutrition, our plates become canvases, painted with the hues of hope and vitality, as we strive to create a future where cancer is met with resilience and triumph.

Chapter Nine

Managing side effects through Nutrition

Imagine a world where each bite is not just a burst of flavor but a powerful ally in the fight against side effects. From the bustling markets of Bangkok to the serene landscapes of Chiang Mai, our culinary expedition introduces a plethora of ingredients renowned for their nutritional prowess. Enter the stage, the mighty turmeric, with its golden glow and anti-inflammatory prowess, curating a medley of dishes that not only soothe but heal.

The delectable dance of coconut milk and lemongrass takes center stage, weaving a tapestry of dishes that promise not just satisfaction to the palate but relief to the weary body. Picture a nourishing Tom Kha soup, brimming with the goodness of coconut, infused with lemongrass, galangal, and kaffir lime leaves – a Thai elixir crafted to ease the side effects of treatment.

As we delve into the heart of Thai cuisine, the vibrant rainbow of fresh vegetables and herbs emerges as a beacon of hope. Enter the world of Pad Thai, where the crunch of bean sprouts and the aromatic basil elevate a simple dish into a nutritional powerhouse, combating fatigue and promoting overall well-being.

But the culinary odyssey doesn't end there – brace yourself for the fiery embrace of chili peppers, not just for their spice but for their potential to alleviate pain and boost the immune system. Picture a Spicy Thai Basil Chicken, a tantalizing blend of heat and healing, offering solace to taste buds and body alike.

In the Cancer Diet Cookbook's exploration of Thai managing side effects through nutrition, we uncover not just recipes but tales of resilience and nourishment. Each dish becomes a chapter, a testament to the healing power ingrained in the rich tapestry of Thai ingredients. So, join us on this culinary adventure where taste and health converge, creating a symphony of flavors that echo the resilience of those embarking on a journey towards wellnes

Chapter Ten

Personal Experience

The author's words mirrored her own struggles, breathing life into the profound emotions that danced within her. The book became a refuge, a sanctuary where she could confront the raw realities of her condition. Each chapter resonated with her, echoing the challenges she faced, and the triumphs she craved. It wasn't merely a collection of words; it was a shared odyssey, a testament to the indomitable human spirit.

As chemotherapy coursed through her veins and uncertainty loomed, the book provided a beacon of understanding. It was a mentor, guiding her through the labyrinth of medical terms and treatment options. In the darkest hours, its narratives served as a lantern, illuminating the path to acceptance and healing.

The author's vulnerability became a source of strength for her, inspiring resilience in the face of adversity. Through her written experiences, she found kinship with others grappling with the same foe. The book was a bridge connecting disparate souls, fostering a community of shared understanding and empathy.

In the silent spaces between medical appointments and restless nights, the author found solace in the rhythmic turning of pages. The prose was a balm for her weary soul, offering not just information but a lifeline to cling to when the currents of despair threatened to pull her under. It became an intimate dialogue, a silent conversation that unfolded as her story intertwined with the author's.

The narrative wasn't just about the struggle against cancer; it transcended the boundaries of illness, delving into the essence of human existence. It painted portraits of courage, love, and the relentless pursuit of life's beauty despite its impermanence. The book was a testament to the resilience of the human spirit, leaving an indelible mark on the author's journey.

As the final chapters of her treatment unfolded, the book stood as a witness to her metamorphosis. It had been a source of wisdom, a companion through the tumultuous storms of uncertainty. Through the author's eloquent prose, the raw emotions of sickness and healing were etched into the pages, creating a narrative that resonated far beyond the realm of her personal experience.

In the end, the book became more than just a guide through illness; it was a beacon of hope, a reminder that even in the face of life's harshest trials, the human spirit could prevail. It was a testament to the transformative power of storytelling, proving that within the written word, one could find not only solace but also the strength to rise from the ashes of despair and embrace life anew.

Conclusion

The cookbook doesn't merely present a collection of recipes; it serves as a compassionate companion on the journey toward better health. By weaving together evidence-based nutritional recommendations and a rich tapestry of flavors, the author not only acknowledges the complexities of cancer treatment but also provides a roadmap for nourishment that extends beyond the confines of conventional dietary guidelines.

The heart of this conclusion lies in the understanding that each recipe is a testament to the author's dedication to offering not just sustenance but a source of comfort and pleasure during a challenging time. The diverse array of nutrient-dense ingredients incorporated into the recipes reflects a commitment to providing a well-rounded and accessible approach to nutrition.

However, the book is not a substitute for personalized medical advice, and the author wisely encourages readers to consult healthcare professionals for individualized guidance. Nevertheless, the meticulous attention to detail in crafting recipes ensures that readers are equipped with a foundation upon which they can build a nourishing diet that aligns with their unique needs.

In essence, "The Cancer Diet Cookbook" is more than a compilation of culinary suggestions; it is a testament to resilience and a celebration of the healing power of thoughtful nutrition. As readers turn the final page, they are left with not just a book but a companion that resonates with empathy and practical wisdom—a guide that empowers them to make informed choices on their journey to well-being.